A FATHER'S TRUE STORY OF HIS A.D.H.D. SON

By

R. A. COLLINS

A
Martal Book
Publication

Martal Book
Publications

This is a First Edition (March 2006)
ISBN 1-903256-32-1

INTRODUCTION

Hello and welcome. First and foremost I would like to thank you for taking the time to read my book. This is the first book I have written, although I have on previous occasions started to write a book only to throw it in the rubbish bin when it is only half completed. This time however, I have actually managed to complete my work, and have it published. The book is only small and I do hope you find it an interesting read. My book is a true story and is based on my own personal experience. It is about a teenager who suffered oxygen starvation at birth, and the subsequent difficulties that followed. You will read about the medical negligence case, the alternative treatments, including acupuncture, homeopathy, faith healing and a visit to the holy waters of Lourdes in France. You will also read about the medication, and the ADHD that John suffers from, along with learning difficulties and autism, with its challenging behaviours. Although each subject will be kept to a minimum, as the extracts are only parts of the book. At first the book may seem to be quite negative but the outcome is fairly positive. I have consulted with John throughout this book and anything he has not been happy with has been left out, the name of the teenager we shall call John, although this is an alias as I considered it to be more appropriate. I have also left out a lot of the extreme behaviours as this subject alone could easily have filled a book. If you have any comments about this book, then I would really like to know, good or bad will be equally appreciated. The purpose of writing about this particular subject is to let it be known what it is like for people with problems such as these, and indeed the carers. Once again thanks and enjoy your read.

If you have any comments please contact my publisher.

THE BIRTH

John is our middle child who was born on the 20th October 1987; this was after being sixteen days overdue. My wife was initially to have a caesarean section according to a doctor she had seen at the outpatients department a week previously and she arrived at the hospital on the 19th October at 8 o'clock, prepared to have her operation. The admitting doctor felt that induction of labour would be impossible because of my wife's obesity, and was of the opinion that a caesarean section would be required. However a decision was made to proceed with induction of labour. At 3.30pm, on the same day of admission, my wife's labour was started off, and after a few problems, the following night at a quarter to one, John was born. John was not breathing and was in a very poor condition, the doctors worked very hard to resuscitate him and after four minutes he was breathing spontaneously. All seemed to be fine and at around 3 o'clock, I headed for home. The following morning I telephoned the hospital and was told that problems had occurred during the night and could I go straight to the hospital, this I did at once and when I saw my wife she was in a distressed state and told me that at 5.45am, a doctor had said to her "your baby is not behaving like a normal baby." During the night John had suffered fits and was in the special care baby unit. I went to see him and it was distressing to see him in such a bad way. On examination in the special care baby unit doctors noted that John was neurologically abnormal, they also suspected that John had septicaemia and a lumbar puncture was performed. This was very traumatic and, according to medical records, contained a large amount of blood. John's kidneys were not functioning, his urine output was almost nil and it was noted to be heavily blood stained and he was given a drug called Manitou to help with this problem. John had actually suffered significant birth asphyxia (Oxygen starvation to his brain), Group B streptococcal septicaemia, epileptic fits, and also kidney failure. To prevent the epileptic fits John was started on a drug called phenobarbatone; this was, at the time, a common treatment for epileptic fits, although I may be right in assuming that newer drugs may be on the market at this time. John was a battler and each day I was seeing improvements in him, how the oxygen starvation was going to affect him was just a matter of waiting. When my wife was discharged John was not well enough to come home and he had to stay in the special care baby unit for some time. When we were able to bring him home we were delighted, we had to give him his phenobarbatone, but this was no big deal. We had many visitors at this time to observe John's health on a regular basis. John astounded the doctors at that time, at how he was progressing after such very serious problems at birth. As John became a little bit older It was clear to me that all was not well and he was diagnosed with ADHD, learning difficulties and challenging behaviours, and later in his life was diagnosed with also being autistic. ADHD is a shortened word for attention deficit hyperactivity disorder, which I will go into later on in my book under the heading of ADHD. I could go on and on about the birth and go into it in a lot more detail but my book is covering a host of different areas, so it is probably time to move on to the next chapter.

THE EARLY YEARS

As soon as John became mobile he was very hyperactive and destructive. At two years old he would climb fences and walls, move the settee and other furniture, and he had an almost obsessive fascination for electrical gadgets, which gave us constant concern for his safety. At this age John had visual problems and this was said to have been a contributory factor to his clumsiness. It is noted in the records of a psychology report that 'John has a severe expressive language delay and visual problems, which undoubtedly contribute to his overall delay. Also extreme behavioural problems, which also may be a contributory factor to his learning difficulties. If given help for these problems his overall potential may well be improved.' John was then referred to behaviour sessions and was seen by a consultant ophthalmologist on the 22nd February 1988. In a letter relating to that visit the ophthalmologists report was as follows, 'He, John, has an atrophic disc on the left and a small pendular nystagmus in that eye only and it is probably seeing very little, if anything at all. The right disc however looks almost normal.' By the time of the review on 11th March 1988, John had made excellent progress; he was growing well and was sitting with support. He was able to roll over unaided and visually appeared to be fixing well, although mild nystagmus persisted in the left eye. At two and a half years of age a report by the speech therapist stated John is presenting with considerable behavioural problems, and subsequently increasing concerns, both about John's language delay and his behaviour problems are voiced in the case notes. In addition the doctor was concerned about John's vision and as a result of the concerns a multidisciplinary assessment was arranged at the hospital. Speech therapy assessment at that time reported, 'John has behaviour control problems and limited attention span, and these are markedly affecting his language development causing it to be delayed and deviant. He rarely interacts, being happy in his own active play. John has no problems with walking, and there is no limitation on the distance that he is able to walk, however he is indeed very clumsy when walking and does tend to bump into things etc., he is prone to spilling drinks knocking over cups of tea or anything in his path. He has an abundance of energy and is able to ride a cycle without stabilisers although he needs to be supervised constantly as he is unsteady and lacks any sense of danger.' At five years old John was unable to dress himself correctly, he would put on his jumper the wrong way round, socks on inside out buttons in wrong holes. John was in nappies until six years old with nappies used at night until he was seven years old, and he was also a very messy eater. A social report stated 'John says that he has many friends at school, but does not have a best friend, and was unable to name any of his friends when I saw him. He is very much a daddy's boy and will give his father a kiss goodnight but not his mother. If John does not get his own way he becomes aggressive and will kick, punch, and break anything that is at hand, in the home or out in the garden.' The report goes on to say that John is very disobedient and does not do anything he is told, his mother is often in tears as this is the most difficult area to deal with. This report was from the social team. When I was at work, my wife would constantly be ringing me up in tears, as it was all too much for her to cope with, especially with another son and daughter to care for, and I would then have to come home. It became so bad that I either had to give up the shop I was running or John would have to go away, I was not willing to let this happen so I decided that I would stay at home and care for John. I would receive a weekly carers allowance. I am told that carers save the government millions of pounds per year, and I suspect this is true. A further report by a consultant paediatric neurologist states, 'John was an extremely active child who was constantly on the go throughout the interview, he did not respond to instruction or suggestion and was not directable at all.' The report goes on to say, 'John presents as a boy with signs of cerebella dysfunction, slightly more marked on the right than the left. He has significant learning difficulties and attention deficit hyperactivity disorder.' The neurologist's prognosis is as follows. 'John is likely to continue to have significant disabilities in the future, his motor deficits are not likely to have a significant impact on his general well being and he is unlikely to be limited to any significant degree by the motor disabilities alone. However he will continue to have general learning difficulties, and the combination of these learning difficulties and his motor difficulties will have a significant impact on his ability to be personally independent. He already requires greater help with certain activities of daily living than might be expected for other children of his age, and it is probable that he will continue to require help and support with some aspects of dressing and personal care in the medium term future, however it is probable that he will become independent in the majority of self care activities with time. It is reasonable to think that John will be unlikely to compete with his peers on an equal basis when he leaves school, and it is probable that he will require much specialised help and advice at that time.' The neurologist adds 'medically John will continue to require input in relation to his ADHD. He is on treatment with Ritalin, which is a stimulant drug used in this condition. This has some associated side effects, which require specialist monitoring and he will need continual reassessment of his requirement for this drug. John's attentional difficulties will probably improve in time but I think he will have significant difficulties with concentration even as an adult. So looking at this report it is obvious to me that John has a long hard struggle ahead and will need all the support he can get.

ABOUT ADHD

ADHD is short for Attention Deficit Hyperactivity Disorder; the symptoms of ADHD are as follows:- Constantly on the go, cannot relax, an abundance of energy, finding it difficult to wait and take turns, short attention span and impulsiveness. John is very impulsive, and on impulse he may just get on his bike and decide to go ten or fifteen miles away from home without telling anyone where he is going. It is not unusual for him to get on a train and go to a town, which may be quite a distance from home. Learning difficulties quite often go in partnership with ADHD, as is the case with John. ADHD individuals tend to chat a lot, and will interrupt others when they are in the middle of a conversation; it is also very difficult for children with this condition to pay attention in a classroom situation. Simple tasks are very difficult to follow. One of the causes of ADHD, according to the medical dictionary, is foetal hypoxia (lack of oxygen to the brain) in the womb or during the birth. Diet does not cause ADHD as some are led to believe, it is possible however that in a few cases it can make the condition very slightly worse, although not of any real significance in the majority of cases. Many studies have shown that diet has no beneficial factors in the attention and impulsivity and also insatiability that are the main problems with ADHD. John takes a Concerta tablet each morning. Concerta is a slow acting Ritalin, which you take once a day and the drug is released slowly into the system throughout the day. The alternative Ritalin needs to be taken two or three times a day. So the slow release is by far the most convenient for the sufferer and carer alike. This medication is one of the stimulant drugs and is proven to be remarkably safe; they have been around for over forty years. These tablets have helped John considerably; we were left with no alternative due to the dangerous situations John was putting himself in. I am convinced, and will always be convinced, that had he not been put on stimulants then by now he would have been killed or very badly injured. In fact one night a young man came to our door in a distressed state, he informed us that John was standing in the middle of the road, in the dark, foggy conditions, with his hands up to stop the traffic. He went on to say he had to swerve and skid to avoid John and he said it was a miracle that he had missed him. This was just one of many such instances. Many people remark, "I would not put my child on these sorts of drugs." I think they should come down to earth and live in the real world. My wife is a diabetic, would I say to her don't take your tablets; let the diabetes kill you instead. ADHD kills and I also think that if it were not for the drugs then the authorities would have taken John away from the family unit. The authorities have in the past suggested this, which is ridiculous, they should try to keep families together by helping with respite, we do not want John away overnight but just a few hours break a week. I also feel that the powers that be were aware of my commitment to keep John at home and that I would strongly fight any drastic measures that were taken to change this. The actual respite we have had over the years has been terrible, even some of the professionals have told us this. I can see very clearly indeed why some families fall apart and I am sympathetic to this, more must be done to help these families who live with so much stress on a daily basis. I will take a quote from the medical dictionary, 'the parents of extremely difficult young children become 'brain dead' and bewildered, they cannot understand why the behaviour regime that works so well for friends and family are so ineffective with their child. They feel criticised by onlookers, friends, and family, they see no easy answers, and they wonder what happened to the joys of parenting. With parents of ADHD children of any age, parents seem to adopt one of three approaches, they accept this temperamental difference, make allowances and parent from the heart, they become overwhelmed feel like failures and lose direction, or they try to drive the bad behaviour out of the child and try to force them to comply.

ABOUT AN ADHD CHILD

You will never force an ADHD child to comply, it is far better to use a more gentle approach. I was in a position with John at a car boot sale one Sunday morning when John was aged around twelve years. A stallholder had a guitar for sale at a price of one hundred pounds, I was not in a financial position to afford it but John wanted it. I said no firmly, John sat on the ground and really hit the roof, a temper tantrum ensued as is common with ADHD. John was behaving uncontrollably, a crowd gathered round and one middle-aged man commented, "what he wants is a bloody good hiding." I thought to myself that's probably what you need, passing such a silly comment without knowing any history of what you see before you. The only way I could calm the situation down was to focus John's mind on something else, i.e. "lets go to the go cart track later." I have been in this position many times, and it would be nice if I was given assistance rather than negative response. Many studies have shown that the stimulant medication is not addictive; we must also never forget that ADHD sufferers tend to suffer from low self esteem, probably due to the fact that they are continually put down, told they are useless and so on. They are also sought out by bullies, as they overreact to taunting, and although they do not start the trouble, they are blamed for the fight that follows. ADHD individuals need to be praised for the positives, this will make them feel good about themselves, thus helping with the self esteem. I have attended many meetings in the past and I never explained how difficult things were as I was afraid that John would be removed from the family unit, the violence was unbelievable, and the tempers were extremely bad. I can put this down now as over the years after a lot of very difficult times, things are improving, albeit slow. The main area of improvement is the tempers. It is estimated that about 1.7 per cent of the population has ADHD. A lot of children who has this condition tend to run away from home, as does John. I have been a regular visitor to the local police station to fill out a missing persons report. Also the local hospital knows us or certainly some of the staff do as we sometimes pay them a visit, normally after John has consumed alcohol in my absence, which is not good if you take the sort of medicine John takes. I am sure that this year since June, we have had to ask for their assistance twelve times and they have been very helpful to the family. Although some children can out grow ADHD it is, on the whole, a lifetime affliction. What I can say with a certain amount of confidence is that as the child grows up and becomes an adult they learn to deal with it in a more positive way in many cases. I strongly believe that even in this day and age, there are individuals in prisons who are afflicted with ADHD and autism, and although have done wrong do not deserve to be in such places, they really needed lots of help prior to offending. It is well documented that ADHD children nag at and demand of their parents from dawn to dusk, this puts enormous pressure on them and generates great tension. A great majority of ADHD children have the social and emotional maturity of other children two thirds of their age. The main treatments for ADHD are advice on behaviour support at school, and indeed the school will need your support, and the use of stimulant medication. The stimulant medication is without doubt the single most effective form of therapy available at this time for the treatment of ADHD. Their has been many studies regarding the benefits of these drugs and it is said that between eighty to ninety per cent will be helped by one of the stimulants in the short term, long term benefits are presumed but not proven. You hear some say natural treatments are safer, but don't you believe it, remember natural does not mean safe as tobacco, opium and magic mushrooms are all natural. I am not saying they are all-bad, in fact I believe they do have a role to play in medicine, and are probably beneficial in a lot of cases. I have outlined the ADHD illness but it is not intended to be an advisory factor, just a small part of my book.

AUTISM
(KANNERS SYNDROME, INFANTILE AUTISM)

This is quoted as a severe psychiatric disorder of childhood, usually with a onset before the age of two and a half years, it is marked by severe difficulties in communicating and forming relationships with other people, in developing language, and in using abstract concepts; repetitive and limited patterns of behaviour and obsessive resistance to tiny changes in familiar surroundings. Autistic children find it very hard to understand how other people feel, and so tend to remain isolated even into adult life. Many are intellectually subnormal, but some are very intelligent and may even be gifted in specific areas, this is the case with John, many have seen the potential that John has, his tutors have informed me of this, and he is truly gifted in certain areas of mechanics especially lawnmowers and the like. The two most import ant causes are genetic factors and brain damage as is in John's case. Treatment for autism is not specific but lengthy specialized education is usually necessary. Behaviour problems and anxiety can be controlled with behaviour therapy and drugs in some cases such as phenothiazines.

The condition of retreating from realistic thinking is a symptom of personality disorder and schizophrenia so you see it is extremely difficult for anyone who suffers with autism.

A BRIEF HISTORY OF A LEGAL CASE

After a normal pregnancy I was a bit concerned as to why John was born with these serious problems, and after very much consideration I decided that I really should try to find out why these problems arose. If I did nothing, would I be acting in John's best interests? I disliked going against the medical profession, but I believe I had to for John's sake. I knew that if I were to go against the might of the health authority then I would need a good legal representative. After much looking around I found a firm of solicitors who were experts in this field. I made an appointment and my wife and I duly met the solicitors. We were greeted warmly and invited into a meeting room, The solicitor was a gentleman of around fifty five years plus, he had a female assistant who, he informed us, was previously a nurse, and was experienced in all aspects of childbirth. My wife gave a detailed account of events and we were in the meeting room for around two hours. We were informed that the next step to be taken was to obtain the medical records from both the hospital concerned and also the family doctor, this would take a while as these procedures quite often do. After going back and forth to the solicitors I was told that I would need to take John to a top London hospital to undergo a specialised MRI scan of his brain, to determine if there was any significant damage to support our case. We received the appointment in due course, and the day came when we were to go. My wife was unable to travel far anymore due to travel sickness and other problems. I travelled with John to London and was surprised that their was no car park, I went to a local council run car park and was flabbergasted to find out that it was to cost me twenty-two pounds to park for the day. We had to park for the day as John was to be sedated for the scan as he would never have been able to lay still long enough for the procedure due to his Attention Deficit Disorder. I went down to the room with John where they sedated him and they put a white fluid into John's vein, and he drifted off, I found this very upsetting as many of you who have witnessed this will understand. I then went for some lunch at a nearby café. On arriving back at the hospital I waited for John to come back, when he did come back we had to wait a while and then John was discharged. We managed to get caught up in all the traffic going home as it was after 5 o'clock. Prior to leaving we were informed that the results would go directly to the solicitors and would take a little while, as they had to be studied very carefully. After a few weeks I was called back to my solicitors to find out the results of Johns brain scan, they were as follows:

Conclusion; the MRI scan shows evidence of end stage infarction. Most such infarcts are due to vascular occlusion for which the aetiology remains uncertain, there is an increased frequency of focal infarction in association with partial hypoxic ischaemia. The time at which the infarct leaving the end stage appearances shown on the MRI scan cannot be determined from the MRI scan appearances alone. However a fairly large infarct occurring after the neonatal period would usually be associated with an acute neurological disturbance. In the absence of any history of such a disturbance it is likely that the infarct took place during the documented period of perinatel illness. Yours sincerely DOCTOR .... F.R.C.R. F.R.C.S. F.R.C.P.

For obvious reasons I am unable to name the doctor who made out this report. There were some aspects of the report which were positive and some not so positive. My next step was to take John to Sheffield to have a report made from a consultant paediatric neurologist, for a file to be prepared for the courts if it proceeded. For the visit to Sheffield I did not want to rely on my old banger of a car so I decided it would be safer to hire a car for this journey. John and I left home at around midday as our appointment was not until 5 o'clock. When we arrived and found the offices, a secretary warmly invited us in and took us through to the specialist. He asked john to do various tasks, and he observed which foot John led with as it can tell an expert a lot. When he had finished his tests we said our goodbyes and then started our journey for home. We were a few miles out of

Sheffield when John started laughing, when I asked him why, he pointed at the car I was overtaking on the motorway. In the car were two policemen and needless to say I didn't really find it that amusing, in any event I was not stopped so I probably was not much over the speed limit, if any. The report I have not been able to find but some parts of the report were quite positive and some were not. A few more months of conferring with solicitors and the time had arrived for me to go to meet with a leading barrister and associates at Crown Office Row in London, to discuss the possible outcome of going to the courts. This time I decided to travel by train as it is sometimes a nightmare driving through the city, John was not required to be present on this trip, which was good, as he would not in any way have been able to sit still throughout the meeting. My appointment was at 5.00 pm which was a peculiar time considering a lot of legal representatives were probably finishing work at that time. When I arrived I was greeted by a very polite, middle-aged lady, who led me into a conference room with about ten professionals seated round a large oval shaped table. A posh coffee pot was on the table along with a tray of biscuits, I felt quite important but found the experience a trifle daunting due to my status compared to theirs. The leading barrister was a portly built man who I would say was probably in his sixties, and I could tell he was a very clever man, indeed he had probably spent the best part of his life in the legal profession, and had probably dealt with many trials of importance. Many venues were explored and pictures of John's brain were on a screen, and I must say I found it difficult to understand a lot of the medical jargon, so found myself asking in layman's terms (what does that mean etc. etc), After much discussion the barrister explained to me that the hospital was almost certainly negligent but it would be extremely difficult to prove that had a different method of birth been tried the outcome would have been any different, and his view was that if the case went to court then it would be a difficult case to win. He reassured me that I had done the correct thing in pursuing the matter, and advised me to act on his advice, which I did. He wished me all the best for the years ahead and hoped that john would improve with the passing of the years. I shook the hands of all concerned and then made my way to the train station, On the train coming home I really did feel quite sad for John due to the negative outcome, but the past is the past and I must put this behind me and move on.

ALTERNATIVE TREATMENTS

I have taken John to a Chinese medicine practitioner, a homeopathic practitioner, and a faith healer. First of all let me tell you about the Chinese medicine. After much research I found a Chinese medicine practitioner who was well recommended. I contacted him to make an appointment, and in due course I took John, with his permission, to see him. On the day we went to see him we were greeted by a small-framed gentleman of Chinese origin, he was polite and reassuring, he took a complete medical history to start with, which took about forty minutes. He then asked John to remove his top and also his socks. He inserted very fine needles in various points on John's body; from time to time he rotated the needles to and fro in a semi circular motion. He never promised any cures or any false hopes, just that he would be willing to give it a try. This treatment, as you may well be aware of, is acupuncture. This traditional Chinese medicine has been around for over 4,000 years and it is a comprehensive medical system with its own principles, diagnostic methods, and therapies. This sort of medicine views the body as an organic whole with a network of meridians connecting and co-ordinating the internal organs, QI [vital energy] blood, body fluids, muscles, bones, tendons, and the skin. Chinese medicine also believe that health in all parts of the body is due to the relative balance of yin and yang, yin yang theory forms the basis of Chinese medicines holistic approach to health and disease, and also offers practical help and guidance in the prevention and management of disease. Acupuncture is used in at least eighty-four per cent of pain clinics in the UK and in primary care for painful and non-painful symptoms. The needles they use are made of stainless steel and are single use disposable needles. Along with the needles the practitioner also used moxibustion with the needles in place, this involves the application of mild heat to the body, again at specific points, with glowing moxa wool [a finely chopped herb folium Artemisia] and this, John told me, was entirely painless. It is essential to find a suitably qualified Chinese herbalist; the register of Chinese herbal medicine association [AACMA] holds lists of practitioners. Go to www. altmedicine.com for further information. We went to the Chinese Medical Centre for about two months and at first it seemed to make John tired and calmer, but the effects were short lived and we saw no significant improvement. So we both came to the decision that we would stop the visits. I believe that Chinese medicine has a big part to play in some conditions, but in John's case it could offer very little. The cost of this treatment was twenty-five pounds per hour with extra money for some herbal tea that John was given.

The next step was to find a homeopathic practitioner to find out what, if anything, they had to offer. Homeopathy is a complementary medicine, which is based on the idea of treating like with like, which aims to stimulate and direct the body's own self-healing abilities. An example of like with like is the Homeopaths remedy Apis Mellifica, which is made from crushed honey bees. It is used to treat medical problems with similar symptoms to the effect of a bee sting, i.e. those that appear suddenly with a severe stinging pain and swelling. There is evidence that homeopathic medicine does work, if you need more information on this the library will have some very useful books on this subject It is said in the medical dictionary that all homeopathic medicines are generally safe, because of the high dilution in which they are used. I found an experienced practitioner of homeopathic medicine and made an appointment. On arriving we were met by a lady of around sixty years of age, she gave me the opinion that she was old fashioned, this was by the clothes she wore, a thick tartan woollen skirt, and the sort of shoes similar to the ones my primary school teacher was often wearing. She knew what she was talking about concerning the homeopathic treatments, I could tell not only by her interpretation of the medicine, but by the huge volume of books on the subject that filled her bookshelves. She took down John's complete medical history, decided on a course of treatment and gave us some tiny white pills of herbal makeup and said to give it a try. After visiting her for a while, I saw no improvements in any way. So again I decided that this would be of no benefit to John and explained to the homeopath that we would no longer be attending. She seemed to be disappointed that the treatment had not been of benefit, and wished John and I all the best. A quote I have taken from the medical dictionary by professor David Peters comments there is no legal regulation of who can call him or herself a homeopath, and therefore it is not always easy to identify a reliable homeopath. Qualifications and registration requirements for homeopaths vary widely between countries, even within the European Union. The UK has no legal regulation of who can practice homeopathy or style themselves a homeopath, and there is no such plans to establish such regulations according to New Medicine 2005. In the UK there are homeopaths that are medically qualified; the faculty of homeopathy is a legal body which trains only registered health professionals. There are also homeopaths who are not medically qualified, if you are considering visiting a suitable homeopath, take recommendations from friends, colleagues, or your family doctor. It is always advisable to ask at the first session about their training registration, experience of treating conditions such as yours and insurances. I felt a little bit sad that the treatments did not help John but I did realise that the possibility was just a shot in the dark. I had taken John to two alternative medical centres and I had one more to visit. This was the one I had no confidence in, but even if the end result was negative at least I tried. The one I am referring to is faith healing; I had heard quite a few tales of the power of prayer now it was time to experience it. I found a faith healer at a healing centre not too many miles from our home, I contacted her and was given an appointment, it was on a Friday night at 5.00. This was a regular time each week. When I arrived with John on our first visit we were greeted by an old lady, who was not a day under eighty years of age, the room smelt very fusty, it was very dull and in a way seemed morbid. The old lady invited us into a room with a bed and a dim light, she asked John to lay down on the bed and relax, this was in itself a major task as John was extremely active at this time. She asked me to hold John's hands and try to keep him still, on the top of the headboard was a wooden cross with a wooden carving of Jesus. The old lady prayed and asked if I could also pray, which I did. On these visits I always saw a young lady, I would say in her early twenties, and she had a very severely disabled boy of about six or seven in her arms, he was both physically and mentally disabled and her appointment was usually after ours, Anyway after a few visits we were able to say without doubt, that this had not helped in anyway, and explained to the old lady that we were not helped and under the circumstances we would end our visits. She said she appreciated our position and would continue to remember us in her prayers. I often wonder what happened to that young boy, and in some ways I do miss seeing him at the centre. There was no charge to go to the healer, but a donation tin was situated on a shelf as you entered the room. On summing up the alternatives, I would say that in our case it did no good. In other cases it may be of benefit, after all even conventional medicine is limited as to what it can offer in cases of brain injury, although things are moving in the right direction, and there is little doubt that in years to come, there will be major advances, especially with stem cell research and also the ongoing research into gene therapy. I would very much like to come back to this planet in about five hundred years time, and if man has not completely destroyed the earth by then. I reckon there will be cures for most diseases and disabilities.

THE LOURDES VISIT

When John was ten years old an opportunity came along for him to go on a pilgrimage to the Holy Place of Lourdes in France; I asked John what he thought about this and he seemed to be quite keen on the idea. A lot of people have no doubt heard of the holy waters of Lourdes, and its miracles that have been said to occur. The story behind it is that of Bernadette. Bernadette Soubirous was fourteen years old, a sickly asthmatic girl in a religious family that had come down in the world, reduced to living in a hovel that had once been a prison cell. On 11th February 1858, Bernadette, her sister and a friend went out to the "old cave" Massabielle, to gather scraps of wood. To reach the spot a shallow canal had to be crossed. Bernadette, worried about her asthma, stayed behind. There, at about 1pm, she felt a warm breeze that seemed to caress her face. Then the vision manifested itself. A 'girl' as Bernadette first described her, spoke kindly in Gascon, telling her "three secrets" and directing her to dig in the cave, where the miraculous spring came forth. Bernadette's talkative sister soon spread the word around and crowds began to gather around the spring. The virgin appeared three more times to Bernadette and too many others as well. By April a kind of hysteria had taken over Lourdes, and miracles could not be far behind. The first was bestowed on Louis Bouriette; blind in one eye, he procured some mud from around the spring, made a compress of it and regained his sight. Newspapers picked up on the story and Lourdes becomes a very busy place. Throughout the carnival that followed, Bernadette seemed to be the only one to keep her head. She continued to have her visions, and described them politely to anyone who troubled to ask; that was all. Bernadette entered a convent up north in Nevers in 1866, where she led a secluded life. Always subject to ill health, she died there in 1879, at the young age of only thirty-five. A movement for canonization sprang up immediately, and in 1933 Bernadette was made a saint. As for her role in history and religion, her own wishes sum it up best, "the less people say about me, the better," she once said. Anyway I decided to let John go on the pilgrimage, as he really wanted to go, and I thought that the experience for him would be a very positive one. Each child had a one-to-one carer who where all very experienced in looking after youngsters with special needs. When the day finally came for John to go, I took him to the venue where he would board the bus. From there they would travel to Dover to cross the English Channel by ferry. I felt quite upset at seeing John leave on the bus, and prayed he would be okay. The trip was fine and everything went according to plan, they did say that John required two carers with him at all times so they had to shift carers around, so that one particular carer was allocated two youngsters who where not quite as active. I witnessed no miracle cures, but was pleased that John had the chance to experience the trip. I cannot go too deeply into the visit to Lourdes as I was unable to go, although no miracles occurred in Johns' case, I feel that he achieved a lot of positive things by going.

EDUCATION

Johns first school was a specialised school who did manage his behaviour quite well, There were many occasions when I did have to pick up John due to the disruptive behaviour he was showing and I remember the assistant in the minibus once securing John to the seat with cord in order to make him sit still. I did not really go along with this approach, but under the circumstances, she may have been correct if she felt that another child in the minibus may have been injured. At five years old John's speech was very difficult to understand, even the school had difficulties in understanding what John he was trying to say. This was very difficult for John and caused him much frustration. John's attention seeking behaviour was also an area of concern, I quote from a school report, 'John's attention seeking behaviour can be distressful to both children and adults alike and results in disappointing poor work on occasions.' The report goes on to say, 'when fully concentrated John is a delightful boy, who is enthusiastic and can produce some really good work. He has made good progress in many areas of the curriculum.' At this school and at John's age he was doing quite well and it was decided to put John in a mainstream school with support. John did not do so well here, and his brother, who attended the same school, was often helping with John, and at the age of around eight years this was not really fair on John's brother. In any event the school could not manage John's behaviour and when the school term ended so did John. It was decided that it would be in John's best interests to let him go back to the first school and so back he went. Again, after a while, it was decided that John attends a mainstream school with support, as he was really doing quite well. I did not really think this was a good move, Things did start to go downhill, and I was often down at the school bringing John home. John could have stayed at his first school until his school days were over, and maybe this would have been the best decision at this point, we will never know for sure, but it seems feasible to me that if a child is doing well at a school, then why the upheaval of moving on to a school where there are good chances of further deterioration. Due to the circumstances the teachers did really well nevertheless and John did have some speech therapy to help him. I remember going to pick John up from a disco at the school, this was prior to John moving on to his final school, he had eaten fourteen burgers a teacher explained to me. This was mostly down to a drug John was on at the time, which made him eat to excess. John felt very sick, "oh, no," I thought, "I hope he does not throw up in the car on the way home." Glad to say he did not and John is no longer on this medication. I could not permit this to continue, and after voicing my concerns to John's psychiatrist he withdrew this horrible drug. A speech therapist's report regarding John's speech was as follows; 'Phonology. This remains John's greatest problem; he can make most speech sounds but continues to have considerable problems sequencing sounds into words, with the result that his speech is often intelligible. He often omits ends of words, and uses a glottal stop in the middle of words. He tries hard but because of his poor attention span, and hyperactivity, there is no long-term consistency of effort and consequently no carry over into speech. He flits from one activity into another, and in spite of long-term speech therapy, progress has been slow and only minimal. I feel his poor attention span and hyperactivity remain a block to his future progress.' The next, and final, school John was to attend was a specialist school, which was a day or a boarding school. John was a day pupil, it would be fair to say for two reasons, John's behaviour and also I preferred John to be at home. The start of the first term was extremely bad. Even John's first day was very bad, after he threw a table in a maths lesson he also provoked a major play-ground fight. A further incident was also quoted in a report, which was extremely serious and resulted in a ten-day exclusion. John was excluded at other times and also on days when I had to go to the school to pick him up due to inappropriate behaviour, which I felt at the time was sometimes out of his control. It has been an extremely difficult task getting John through his school years, and there is light at the end of the tunnel.

I have supported him all the way. I have not missed any of his sports days, reviews and Christmas concerts. In fact because of my commitment to John my other children have been left out, and indeed missed out on a large majority of their childhood, but this is a well recognised fact which is without any doubt. John has left school now, but still attends a unit in the grounds where he is doing some college work with a tutor, and he is making remarkable progress. He also spends one day a week at an establishment gaining work experience. He has gone from being absolutely uncontrollable to a person who has so much to give, he also helps a man and his wife, who live a short distance from our home, with gardening and odd jobs etc., which he enjoys and also the people enjoy his company.

THE DRUGS

John takes three different medications, the first one I will mention is the Melatonin. This is the all-natural nightcap. Melatonin is produced normally in the brain, it is just that John needs a little bit more to help him wind down and get to sleep. What melatonin does is to help with the sleep-wake cycles by being released at night in order to help you sleep. As we get older our bodies do not need as much Melatonin and as a result less is produced. Scientific studies suggest that Melatonin can hasten sleep without the hazards or side effects of many of the prescription sleeping pills. It also may have many other uses, current research is underway to find out Melatonin's effect as an anti-oxidant, delayed sleep phase disorders, and also jet-lag. It is stated that there is still much to be learned about Melatonin and its benefits on the human body. Tests on laboratory mice suggest that it can reduce the effects of aging, but remember these are only preliminary. Also there are some people who should avoid taking Melatonin and they are pregnant women, people with severe allergies and people with auto-immune diseases. It is also recommended that woman trying to conceive should think twice about taking Melatonin as in high doses it is said to possibly act as a contraceptive. Is it safe; Melatonin is one of the least toxic substances known, the only evidence is that in high doses it may possibly cause drowsiness and slower reaction times. In the USA melatonin is readily available over the counter. John only takes a minimum dose at night, as this is the time it should be taken if you have sleep problems. Natural, animal or bovine grade Melatonin comes from animal tissue, and this sort of Melatonin may be accompanied by viruses or proteins that can cause an antibody response, it is highly recommended that people stay away from it. The alternative, which is what John takes, is synthetic or pharmacy grade Melatonin. This is produced from pharmaceutical grade ingredients, and this Melatonin is molecularly identical to the Melatonin we produce in our bodies without the unwanted extras. The actual dose John takes of Melatonin is six milligrams per night. One of the other drugs that John takes is Olanzapine (Zyprexa) this belongs to a group of medicines called antipsychotics, and is used for diseases with symptoms such as hearing, seeing, or sensing things which are not there, mistaken beliefs, unusual suspiciousness, and becoming withdrawn. It is also used to treat a condition with symptoms such as feeling high, having excessive amounts of energy, needing much less sleep than usual, taking very quickly with racing ideas and sometimes severe irritability. It is also a mood stabiliser that prevents further occurrences of the disabling high and low (depressed) extremes of mood associated with this condition. John is on the lowest dose possible of Zyprexa 2. 5 mgs. They start at this dose and then there are 5mgs 1, 5mgs.1 0mgs, 15mgs. and 20mgs. Like all medicines Zyprexa can have side effects but to date John has not suffered any noticeable effects, and I do hope it will continue. The third and final medication John takes is the drug I have already mentioned called Concerta XL (Ritalin) This is a prolonged release tablet, this means that they release the active ingredient slowly, the outer layer of the Concerta XL tablet dissolves right after it is swallowed in the morning, giving your child an initial dose of methylphenidate. The tablets have a special membrane that enables the rest of the methylphenidate to be released from the tablet at a gradual rate following the delivery of the initial dose from the outer layer. The tablet does not dissolve completely after all of the drug has been released and sometimes the tablet shell may appear in the stools, this is perfectly normal. John does not suffer any significant side effects from taking Concerta XL. The benefits he gets from the drugs are enormous and have indeed helped him in his life in a variety of ways. So ends my description of the drugs.

IMPACT ON FAMILY

As some readers may be aware, if you have a family member that suffers with ADHD, the effects on the rest of the family are devastating. The brothers and sisters live a completely different lifestyle than in a normal family surrounding, they have to witness the terrible temper tantrums, the bad language, the police visiting our home, the times when we go out as a family and we all have to come home early due to some problems that John has given us. We have been on holiday in a chalet and John has run away somewhere, and half the night has been spent looking for him, after three or four nights you really have had enough and we pack up and head for home. This affects the other children. I remember in our previous house we only had two bedrooms upstairs and one room downstairs that we used as a bedroom, the two boys were together, as this was the only way we could arrange it as our daughter had one of the upstairs bedrooms, and on a nightly basis it caused problems as John did not sleep until around one o'clock, he was noisy and this started fights between the two boys, and as a result I was forever up and down the stairs, I really did feel very desperate. We moved to a larger house and this did help with the sleeping arrangements. During John's temper tantrums he would lash out at all of his family, during one of the episodes he hurt his sister and she told her teacher what had happened. I was called to the school and after talking to the teacher it was decided to try to resolve the matter within the family, had the authorities been involved it most certainly would have been a very serious situation. It must also be born in mind, that other children in the family get remarks thrown at them which can be hurtful i.e. your brother is stupid. Sometimes words have been said to John's sister that I could not possibly put in print. We have had a lot of professional involvement over the years to assist with John's problems and this can make the other children feel left out. As a further consequence it is a fact well documented that brothers and sisters fall behind with their schoolwork, parents also suffer with health problems, I have been suffering with blood pressure for the last few years and I do have palpitations on almost a daily basis. Stress is the suspect cause, I have been on a heart machine a few times and it did not show anything sinister, however I am convinced that my lifespan will be reduced because of the stress over the years. I know of families who have been parted because of all the stress involved, as it is difficult to work together in a lot of circumstances, in the past my wife has made it quite clear that she would prefer John to go somewhere residential as the strain has been to much, and most of the time in the past this was our main disagreement, nevertheless we have seen it through and have stuck together, of which we feel proud. Many times I personally have been told things such as "you will never do anything with John" also remarks such as "the best thing is to put John in some residential settings," we all know what is best if it is not our child don't we? These remarks made me more determined than ever and in an odd sort of way spurned me on. We understand the need for professional involvement, and some have been supportive, some have not, in as much as some of the authorities who were on many occasions due to turn up at meetings did not turn up, and made no apologies, and the particular authority which was really crucial in supplying respite, which we have had very little of due to funding. Even many of the professionals involved have raised this point at many meetings, confirming how we have been let down by the system. I really think that behaving well towards people with learning difficulties should be a quite important part of the school curriculum, as it can and does affect many people's lives, not just the afflicted.

JOHN'S ACHIEVEMENTS

Johns achievements have been quite remarkable considering, and the future for John is looking far better than could have been imagined a couple of years ago. John is doing a college course, and has an entry level certificate for mathematics, (entry 3), which is the highest level of award for an entry certificate, he also has an entry level certificate for English, (entry 2), and further more has an entry level certificate for physical education, again the highest level of award for an entry level certificate, (entry 3). John has swimming certificates and is indeed a very strong swimmer, last summer we went to the coast and I said we could not go into the sea as it was extremely rough, John ignored my pleas and went straight in, he swam like a fish. A man on the beach said to me "you wouldn't get me out there today and I consider myself to be a strong swimmer." I kept on shouting to John to come out of the water but I may as well have been speaking to a brick wall. John also has his cycling certificate. Although John is doing a college course it is within a school in a unit with a tutor, he also attends a gardening establishment as part of his work experience, he is very good at repairing lawn mowers, and this is his main hobby. This keeps John occupied as he needs to be doing something all the time, otherwise he gets bored. He has a small workshop at home and a few mowers, so if you have any old mowers or mechanical items that you no longer need and intend dumping them, please consider letting John have them to gain experience. John is one of three students on a college course, an individual special programme for students with exceptional complex needs. John has settled well into his course. It is his tutor's view that John could work to GCSE level on this subject. John travels a fifty-mile trip daily to his college course and he does not mind it, in fact I believe he quite enjoys it. He has been on two trips to France in total, once as explained to Lourdes, and again with a school trip. He has been on various cycling trips with other youngsters and his tutor, and has also participated in some charity events. His next big aim is to get a licence to drive a car, and although it is difficult for John to get a licence at this moment in time, due to his medical problems, I think that one day, if things keep going the way they are then it would be a strong possibility, I shall support John with this when the time is right. I would be surprised if he does not continue improving now that things have started to move in a positive direction. I think that John has, and will, achieve much more in his life. John says that he would like his own place to live, and we are looking into this at the moment, we have been told by people helping us with this that the local council has places that are warden controlled, this may be the answer, but we feel strongly that John is not ready as yet to live an independent life. Again we will support him all we can at the appropriate time. We trust John enough now to let him go to a local nightclub, something we would not even been able to consider a short time ago, the nightclub owners are aware of John's difficulties and they do keep a watchful eye on him as much as is possible, at the end of the day I would prefer John not to go, but you really have to give these kids a chance, after all they do not normally start any trouble, it is usually because of their vulnerability that they tend to get picked on by a minority, and I mean a minority, most of the youngsters are good sensible kids who do understand. A lot of the kids in the small town know John and are really good, they even take the time and trouble to ring me up if John is in trouble, thank God of late they have had no reason to ring me up, long may it continue.

MORE NEEDS TO BE DONE

Much more needs to be done to help all people with learning difficulties, more social clubs are needed along with more specialized sheltered housing accommodation. I also have read many cases in the media about people with learning difficulties who have either peen subjected to the most horrific of beatings, or have been robbed or even murdered by the scum of society. Is the system failing these folks, are sentences too soft, I personally know a chap who I became quite fond of many years ago after he regularly came into the shop I was running at the time, he had quite severe learning difficulties but was far more intelligent than people thought, and he came into my shop one day with two black eyes. It came to light that he had been beaten up, I just could not believe it, how could someone do this to another human being let alone a vulnerable member of society. I wonder sometimes if man really does have the right to exist on this planet Earth. My way of thinking is not merely because I have a member of my family effected by learning difficulties, I would still feel the same way under any circumstances. So I do think that it is extremely important that respect for all people should be a quite serious issue as far as the school curriculum is concerned, it should be taught on a weekly basis. All people have the right to be respected, no matter what colour, race, status etc., there is nobody any better than anyone else we are all equal. I am no better than a tramp and a king is no better than I. The main areas that I consider where more needs to be done are as follows -

(1) Education many youngsters who have learning difficulties miss out on a decent education, I have witnessed this first hand, and have seen many more cases in the media, it is very important that these people get off on the right note by having a decent education. Many youngsters are excluded due to inappropriate behaviour time after time after time, you cannot put the blame on the teachers, it goes beyond that. The schools especially the special schools should have far more support to help with difficult pupils.

Also it is often recommended that children attend schools many miles from their homes with the only alternative to stay away for a week at a time, or sometimes longer. Many parents do not allow this and as a consequence the child misses out on education or, in a worse case scenario, risks prosecution by the education authorities. Mainstream schools are normally within a short distance from the pupils home so the pupils are home each day, I believe this should be the same for learning disabled children, could not all schools have special units with specialised teachers to assist. I must admit I am not sure if this would work but what is the answer.

(2) Housing. This is a very important area and quite often needs the help of professionals experienced in this field. You do not just give people with learning disabilities a flat, house, or whatever and leave them to get on with it, many issues need to be considered depending on the individual. Many need support, which is ongoing such as warden assisted, or a carer, or perhaps some other form of assistance. Without a secure base the results are without any doubt disastrous. I still feel that many of these vulnerably people without a permanent home finish up in jail, or on drugs, prostitution, the list goes on. Should vulnerable people be in the main *type* of prison, I think not, my opinion is that there should be a complete review of the prison service, and anyone suffering from these illnesses should be moved to a more appropriate surrounding.

SUMMARY

I think that the most worrying aspect of having a person in your family who has challenging behaviours is the attitudes of some individuals, at least this is what I have experienced throughout the years, especially with people knocking at the door, saying John has done this, John has done that, also picking John up from hostile situations. I can say without doubt that since John came along I am a much more understanding person, and can indeed relate to others in a similar situation. I feel that I am a much better person inside and I tend not to make a lot of fuss over the minor things in life. I have attended many functions for youngsters with learning disabilities, and I always feel so very sad, but I am always astounded, by their outlook and achievements. I hope that the contents of the book have not offended anyone, if so please accept my most sincere apologies, once again thanks.

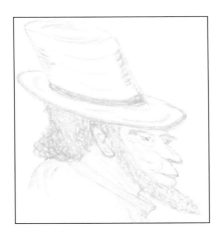

For further information about this
or any of our publications, please
contact Martal Publications of Ipswich

Customer Helpline 01473 720573
Email: martalbooks@msn.com

Published and Printed
by
Martal Publications of Ipswich
PO Box 486
IPSWICH
United Kingdom
IP4 4ZU